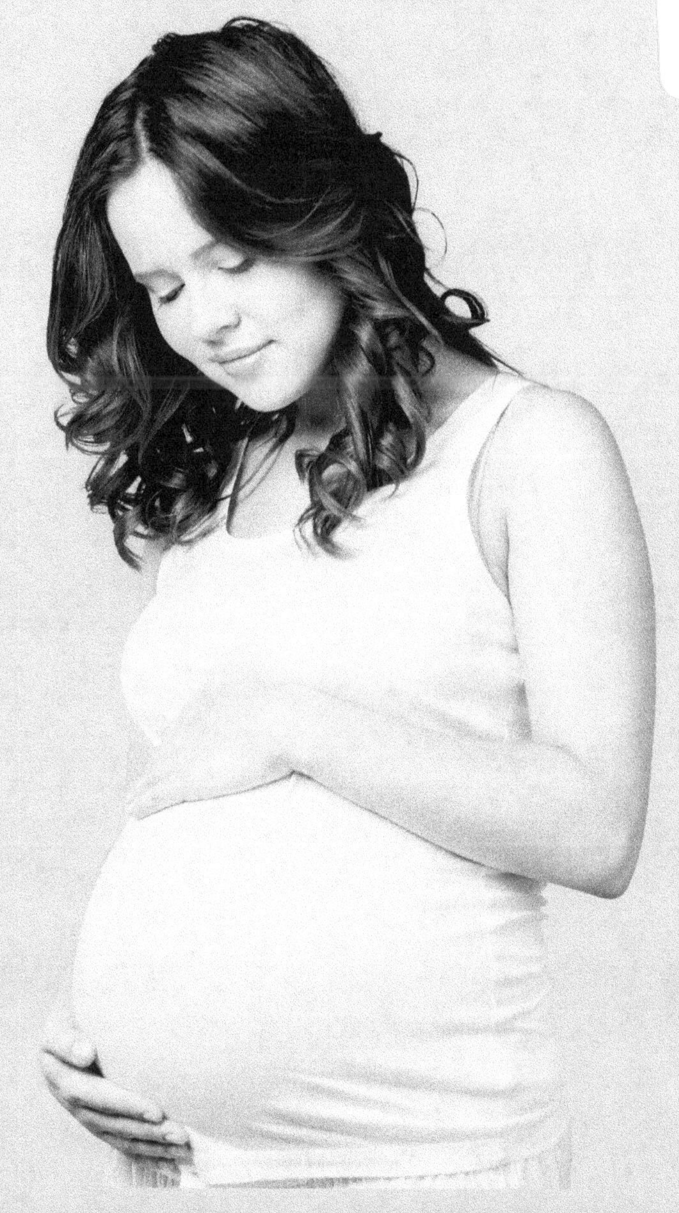

FITNESS AND NUTRITION DURING AND AFTER PREGNANCY

BEN JOHN

DISCLAIMER

All the material contained in this book is provided for educational and informational purposes only. This material should not be considered a substitute for professional medical advice, diagnosis or treatment.

The author has made every effort to ensure the accuracy and practicality of the information provided in this book but assumes no responsibility for errors or inappropriate use of the information.

Printing this book will make it easier for you to read.

This information is provided as a courtesy and you are free to use it but not obligated.

FITNESS AND NUTRITION DURING AND AFTER PREGNANCY

CONTENTS

CHAPTER 1

INTRODUCTION

FITNESS AND NUTRITION DURING AND AFTER PREGNANCY

INTRODUCTION

For many women, becoming pregnant and giving birth are among life's greatest miracles. When asked what the most memorable event in their lives was, many people cite pregnancy or parenthood as an answer—or both!

In the face of such strong emotions, it is impossible to deny that pregnancy and childbirth are a gift.

While pregnancy can be a beautiful and rewarding process, the unpleasant reality is that eating well and getting regular exercise are both important during this time.

However, there is a downside to this rosy picture. Many women feel that pregnancy has ruined their figure and made them unattractive due the stretch marks it leaves behind—despite not having gained much weight at all (or even losing some).

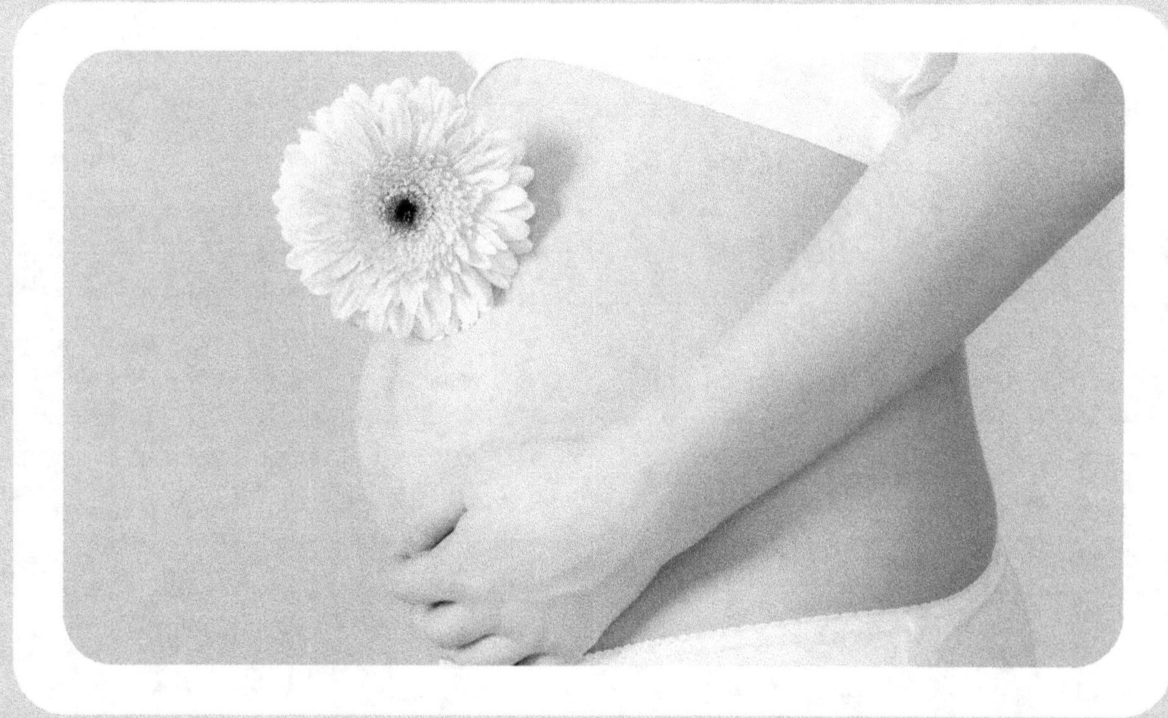

Many women believe that after they give birth, their bodies will never return to the size and shape they used to have. They consider weight gain, stretch marks and a loss of sexual appeal as negative consequences of having a bouncy little baby—trade-offs.

This could not be farther from the truth.

Yes, pregnancy will result in weight gain. But that doesn't mean you have to let yourself go—you can keep the pounds off without much trouble.

All weight gain in pregnancy is eventually lost. It may seem impossible to lose the extra pounds during or after pregnancy, but it's a matter of knowing how and having patience with yourself as you work toward your goal.

It will take time to shed the fat you gained during pregnancy—but that's okay. Slow and steady wins the race, or so they say! With patience and persistence, you can definitely lose excess weight after having a baby.

You can become fitter and stronger after childbirth if you work hard enough at it. Your body will adjust to the demands of motherhood as readily as to changing weather conditions or an increase in workload at work.

What truly matters is that you believe the change in your body composition can be achieved. You must release false beliefs that pregnancy and childbirth will result in an unattractive woman.

During pregnancy, your body makes extra blood and stores fat for breast milk. After childbirth, these changes reverse themselves so that you will lose weight.

Even the world's most famous female celebrities have expressed their own personal struggles with weight gain during pregnancy.

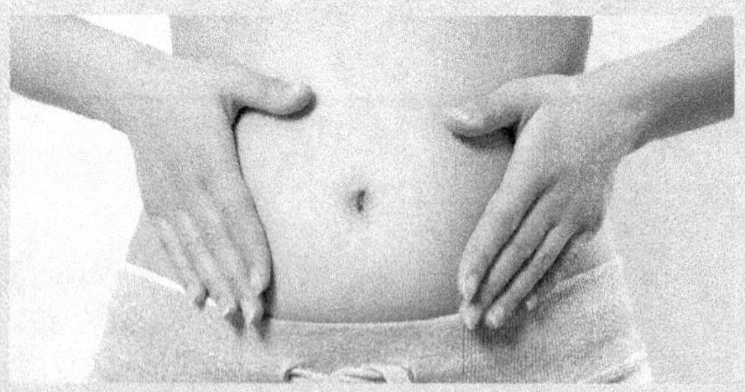

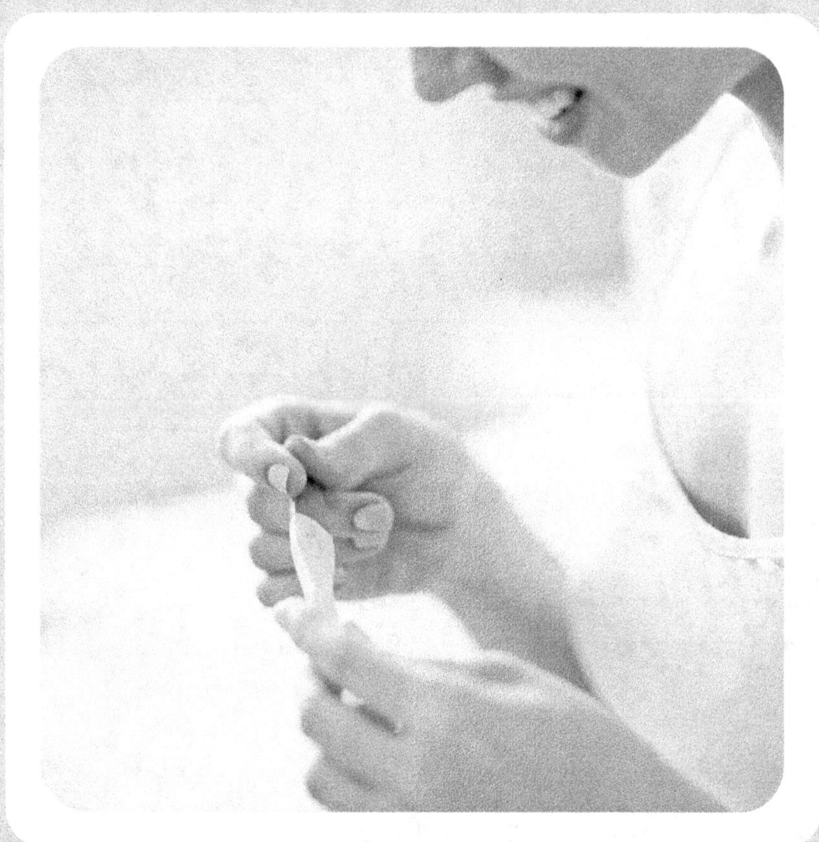

It is normal to gain weight and it takes time to lose it. You will feel down at times during your journey, but don't let that discourage you from making progress every day.

Yes, it will be hard. But you can do it! Losing weight after childbirth is only one aspect of the long-term process of changing your body and self-image.

This book will help you understand and implement the necessary changes for achieving your pregnancy, birth and postpartum goals.

You will only reap the benefits of this book if you take its advice and apply it to your life.
During your pregnancy, you'll need to know how to eat well and stay physically active. You may also want to consult a doctor or nutritionist about supplements that are safe during pregnancy.

This book will help you understand and implement the necessary changes for achieving your pregnancy, birth and postpartum goals.

You will only reap the benefits of this book if you take its advice and apply it to your life.

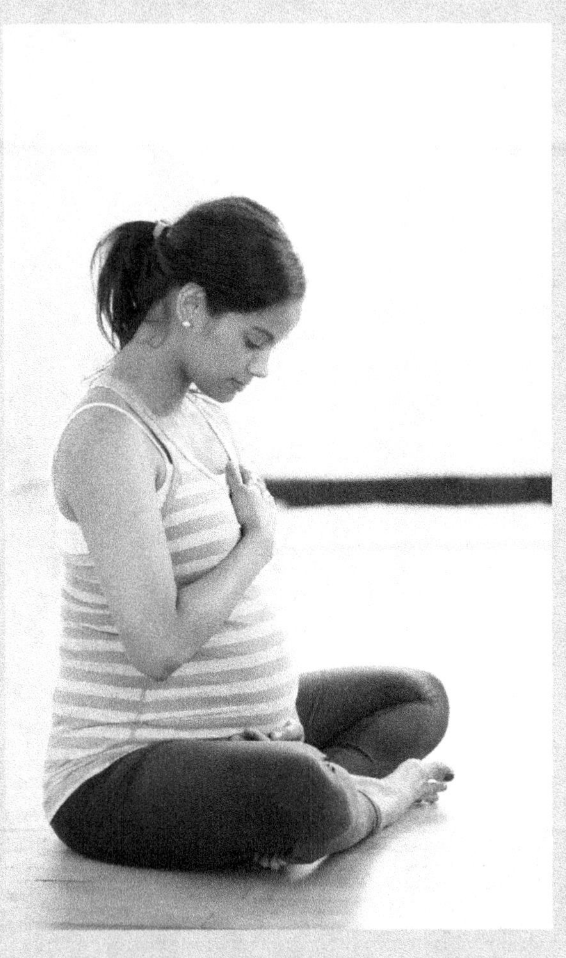

You can become fitter and stronger after childbirth if you work hard enough at it. Your body will adjust to the demands of motherhood as readily as to changing weather conditions or an increase in workload at work.

What truly matters is that you believe the change in your body composition can be achieved. You must release false beliefs that pregnancy and childbirth will result in an unattractive woman.

During pregnancy, your body makes extra blood and stores fat for breast milk. After childbirth, these changes reverse themselves so that you will lose weight.

Even the world's most famous female celebrities have expressed their own personal struggles with weight gain during pregnancy.

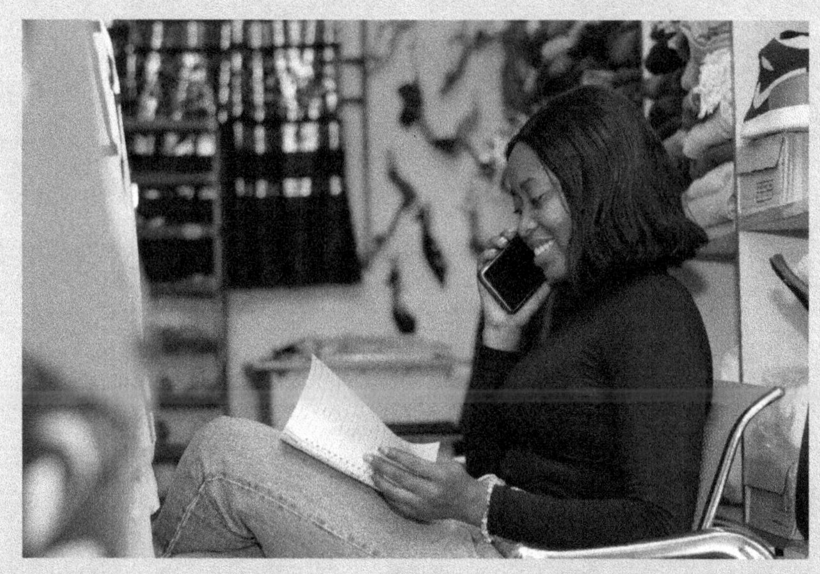

CHAPTER

2

WHAT EVERY PROSPECTIVE PARENT NEEDS TO KNOW!

FITNESS AND NUTRITION DURING AND AFTER PREGNANCY

Before you even get pregnant, understanding how your health, habits, diet and fitness level affect fetal development can help you live a healthy life during pregnancy.

Smoking during pregnancy can cause a lot of damage to both the mother and her child.

If you plan to get pregnant, you must eliminate any negative habits before conception.

Ideally, you should exercise regularly and eat healthfully before trying to get pregnant. You should also give up smoking, drinking alcohol or doing anything else that might harm your baby-to-be.

Proper nutrition is important at all stages of a person's life, including during the pre-conception and pregnancy periods.

Your baby is completely dependent on you for food and other necessities. It makes sense that you would want to give your child the best possible start in life—the kind of nutrition found only in breast milk.

A fetus shows no visible signs of malnutrition during your monthly check-ups. Even a doctor would have difficulty determining whether the baby is getting all its nutrients.

In order to ensure the health of both yourself and your baby, you will have to eat enough for two people and make sure that you get all the necessary vitamins and nutrients. Only by being proactive in this way can you keep your family healthy.

Here are some tips if you're trying to get pregnant.

- **NO SMOKING & NO ALCOHOL**

  No negotiation here.

- **CONSUME 400 TO 800 MICROGRAMS (400 MCG OR 0.4 MG) OF FOLIC ACID EVERY DAY.**

  You should talk to your doctor about this. Your physician can help you decide how folic acid affects neural tube defects during pregnancy.

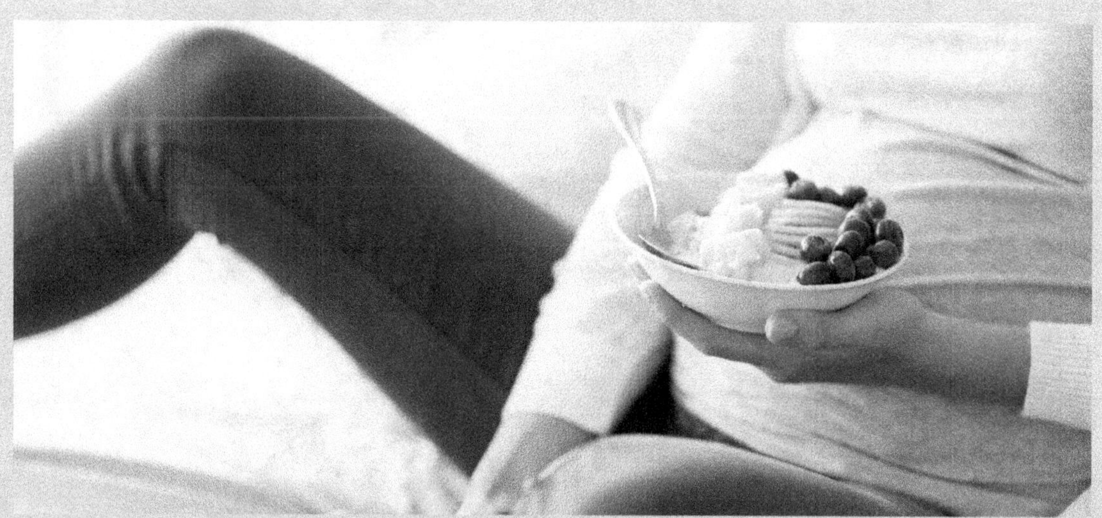

- **MAKE OTHER HEALTH PROBLEMS A PRIORITY**

  If you have any health problems, such as diabetes or asthma, get them under control before trying to conceive.

- ### **GET FIT AND HEALTHY**

  Exercise more to build up your strength, stamina and endurance. When you're pregnant, it will be easier on both you and the baby if you can manage physical activities without getting excessively tired or out of breath.

- ### **ASK YOUR PARTNER TO BE ACTIVELY INVOLVED**

  If your partner continues to smoke or engage in other activities that are harmful, they should try and stop for the sake of the baby.

  At the very least, if they can't quit, they shouldn't smoke around you or tempt you by consuming alcohol around you.

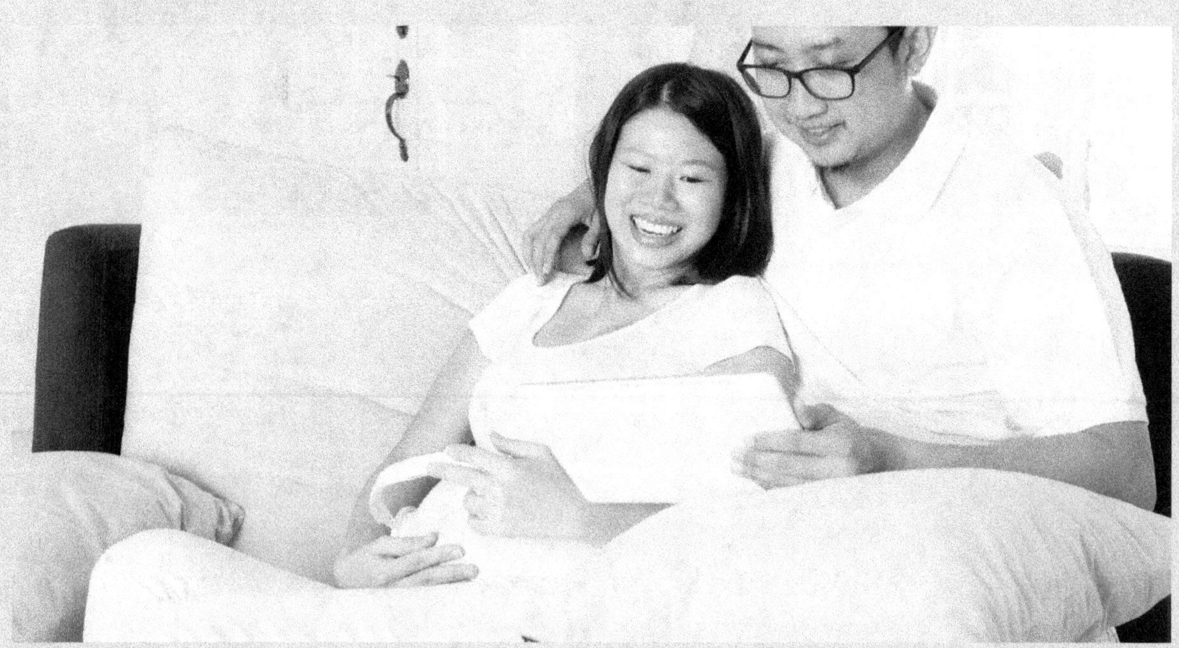

CHAPTER 3

NUTRITION AND FOODS THAT ARE BEST FOR PREGNANCY HEALTH

The ancient Greek physician Hippocrates said that food could be used as medicine, and medicines should also be eaten.

You'll feel much better physically and emotionally if you eat well during your pregnancy.

Our society is drowning in a sea of food options, but most of these choices are unhealthy.

Additives, preservatives and chemicals are found in processed foods. Junk food is high in calories but low in nutrients. Genetically modified organisms can be harmful to the environment.

An epidemic of obesity has plagued the nation, with diabetes and other related diseases escalating dramatically. The cause is clear: our increasingly sedentary lifestyle and poor eating habits.

Eating clean and losing weight takes time. It can't happen overnight, and willpower alone won't make it happen.

You should start making these changes gradually before you become pregnant so that it becomes a habit.

You can transition from a high-fat diet to one that is low in fat a little easier by taking it slowly.

HOW MANY CALORIES DO I NEED TO CONSUME?

Many women find themselves caught in this dilemma: they don't want to consume too many calories, but then sudden food cravings pop up and seem to come out of nowhere.

A pregnant woman should not obsess over calories. She should focus on eating well-balanced meals because her fetus is growing quickly and needs a lot of nutrients for growth.

While pregnancy gives you permission to not count calories for 9 months, it's important not to gorge on whatever food comes your way.

A pregnant woman should not obsess over calories. She should focus on eating well-balanced meals because her fetus is growing quickly and needs a lot of nutrients for growth.

Eat the right amount of food to avoid undernourishment, but don't starve yourself.

A mother's poor diet often contributes to low birth weight, poor fetal development, and weakness. Take into account that pregnancy weight gain is temporary, and be determined to work off what you add during your nine months.

Consuming too many calories can cause you to gain weight and put you at risk for diabetes, heart problems and other medical conditions.

It's important to eat enough for your own body, but it's also essential that you nourish the baby.

Before you figure out how many calories your body needs to maintain its current weight during pregnancy, you will need to calculate the number of calories it would have needed if you weren't pregnant.

Here are some foods you should eat while pregnant. Although they're healthy for anyone, these choices can benefit an unborn baby as well.

You're more aware of the role food plays in your life, and that's because there is an actual living being inside of you who will grow up depending on what you put into his or her body. And yes, this responsibility can feel a little intense at times.

FOODS YOU MUST EAT

In the fitness industry, there is a saying that "a calorie is not created equal."

If you consumed 300 calories of bananas and apples, the results would be different from those produced by eating all 300 calories in the form of ice cream.

Will the benefits be the same? Based on your answer, which food would you choose for your baby?

For example, broccoli would be considered a single ingredient food. Since the only ingredients you need to make broccoli are water and dirt, it is classified as an extremely basic form of produce.

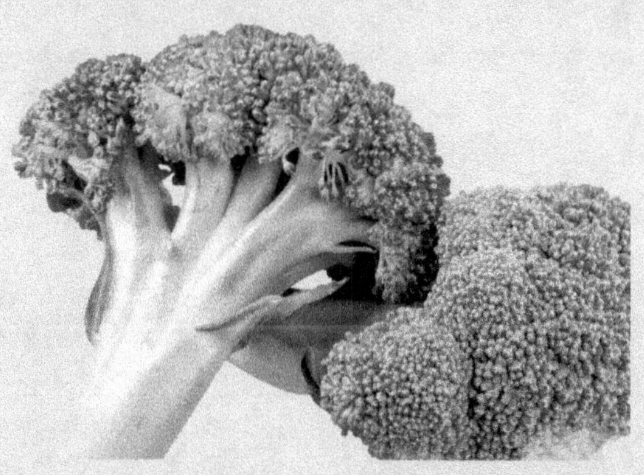

WHITE BREAD

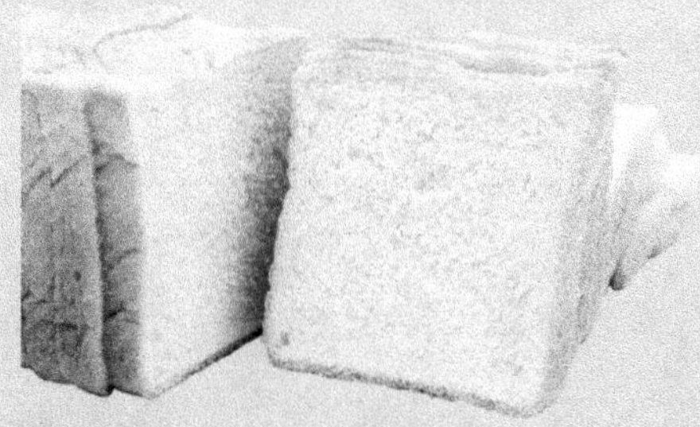

Most people don't know how it's made, what ingredients are used, or how to make their own bread as white.

If you do not know what is in a food, it's better to avoid it. White bread often includes refined flour that has been bleached white and contains all kinds of artificial ingredients.

Processed foods are bad for your body. Eat natural, simple food instead.

EAT FRUITS AND VEGGIES

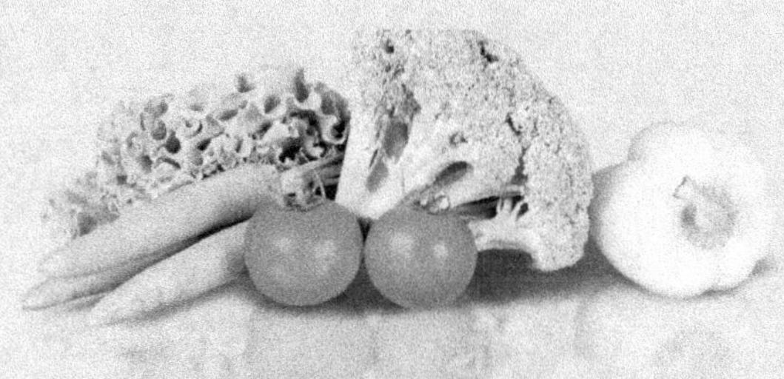

We all know that fruits and vegetables contain a ton of vitamins and minerals that are essential to our health. If you want to be healthy, eat these every day (and make sure they're organic!).

Eating an apple every day can help keep a person healthy.

If you're going to build something meaningful in your life, it takes time. There are no shortcuts.

While carbohydrates have gotten a bad rap over the years, they are essential to our health in many ways. In particular, carbs provide energy and are integral to your daily calorie needs while pregnant.

It's important that you choose carbs wisely. Fruit, vegetables, and whole grain loaves of bread (and the like) are all excellent carb sources.

White bread, pasta and other products made from white flour are bad carbohydrates.

TRY AND KEEP IT ORGANIC IF POSSIBLE

Lean meats, eggs, beef and beans are great sources of protein. Be sure to choose only those that have a single ingredient (e.g., chicken breast rather than nuggets).

While eating organic foods can be more costly, it is highly beneficial for pregnant women to consume organically grown food.

Organic foods are produced without the use of synthetic pesticides or fertilisers.

If you cannot afford to buy all of your organic food, then at least buy some organic foods.

The Environmental Working Group, a non-profit organisation that studies the effects of pesticides on human health and well-being, has found high levels of certain harmful chemicals in many fruits and vegetables. Therefore you should try to keep these organic whenever possible: apples, bell peppers, celery cherries, grapes, nectarines, peaches, pears, spinach strawberries.

EAT THE RIGHT KIND OF FAT

Extra virgin olive oil and virgin coconut oil are both good types of fat to consume, but the latter is better.

Typically, saturated fat is found in animal products such as butter. These forms of saturated fats are best eaten in moderation.

If you are unsure what to eat and drink, follow this menu.

VITAMINS	FOOD SOURCE
Vitamin A	Liver, carrots, sweet potatoes, kale, spinach, collard greens, cantaloupe, eggs, mangos and peas
Vitamin B6	Fortified cereals, bananas, baked potatoes, watermelon, chick peas and chicken breast
Vitamin B12	Red meat, poultry, fish, shellfish, eggs and dairy foods
Vitamin C	Citrus fruits, raspberries, bell peppers, green beans, strawberries, papaya, potatoes, broccoli and tomatoes
Calcium	Dairy products, fortified juices, fortified butters and fortified cereals, spinach, broccoli, okra, sweet potatoes, lentils, tofu, Chinese cabbage, kale and broccoli.

VITAMINS	FOOD SOURCE
Vitamin D	Milk, fortified cereals, eggs and fatty fish (salmon, catfish and mackerel)
Vitamin E	Vegetable oil, wheat germ, nuts, spinach and fortified cereal
Folic Acid	Oranges, orange juice, strawberries, leafy vegetables, spinach, beets, broccoli, cauliflower, peas, pasta, beans, nuts and sunflower seeds
Iron	Red meat and poultry, legumes, vegetables, some grains and fortified cereals
Vitamin B3	Eggs, meats, fish, peanuts, whole grains, bread products, fortified cereals and milk
Protein	Beans, poultry, red meat, fish, shellfish, eggs, milk, cheese, tofu, yogurt, fortified cereal and protein bars
Riboflavin	Whole grains, dairy products, red meat, pork, poultry, fish, fortified cereals and eggs
Thiamin	Whole grains, pork, fortified cereals, wheat germ and eggs

VITAMINS	FOOD SOURCE
ZINC	Red meats, poultry, beans, nuts, grains, oysters, dairy products and fortified cereals

SUPPLEMENTS BEFORE, DURING AND AFTER PREGNANCY

FITNESS AND NUTRITION DURING AND AFTER PREGNANCY

Food alone cannot provide your body with all the necessary nutrients, vitamins and minerals.

A varied diet with nutrition knowledge is necessary to ensure a completely balanced diet without any nutritional deficiencies.

Most women don't have time to watch their diets like hawks and note everything they consume. Taking supplements can help make up for the vitamins you miss out on by not eating well.

Although you might be tempted to skip the nutrition part of your pregnancy, because it sounds overwhelming or confusing, basic knowledge about what you should eat and why can make all the difference.

There is a list further down with 14 important supplements you should consume. Do note that the Recommended Daily Allowances are just a rough estimate. Speak to your doctor and tailor your supplement intake to best suit your needs.

One thing you should know is that there are negative effects of overdosing on certain vitamins. This usually occurs when a person eats foods containing a particular vitamin and also takes supplements of that vitamin. Now the body has more than it needs, so something bad happens (such as an illness or deficiency in another nutrient).

One of the ways that you can protect your baby is to share with your doctor what you're eating and any vitamins, medications or supplements (including herbal) that you're taking during pregnancy.

They will assess your diet by asking questions about how you eat. Be sure to answer every question, no matter how unimportant it may seem.

These are the supplements that I recommend.

VITAMIN A

Vitamin A is essential for the development of a baby's bones, teeth, heart, ears and eyes. Its role in helping the immune system function properly cannot be overstated.

Vitamin A is essential in small amounts, but if taken in too-large quantities can cause birth defects and liver toxicity. Do not exceed 3,000 mcg (10,000 IU) per day.

Vitamin A can be found in liver, carrots, sweet potatoes, kale, spinach collard greens, cantaloupe, eggs, mangos and peas.

VITAMIN B6

Vitamin B6 is a water-soluble vitamin that aids in the development of the baby's brain and nervous system. It also encourages the growth of new red blood cells in both mother and child. Some women report that B6 has helped alleviate their morning sickness.

A pregnant woman and her nursing infant should consume at least 1.9 mg of vitamin B6 daily. That amount rises slightly when nursing to 2.0 mg per day.

Vitamin B6 is found in fortified cereals, bananas, baked potatoes, watermelon and chickpeas. Chicken breast is also a source of the vitamin.

VITAMIN B12

Vitamin B12 and folic acid work together to produce healthy red blood cells and promote the development of a healthy brain and nervous system in the baby.

Most people have sufficient stores of vitamin B12, and it is very rare to suffer from a B12 deficiency.

According to the Office of Dietary Supplements, pregnant women should consume at least 2.6 micrograms (104 IU), and nursing mothers 2.8 micrograms (112 IU) of vitamin B12 daily.

It can be found in a variety of foods, including red meat, poultry, fish, shellfish, eggs and dairy products.

VITAMIN C

Vitamin C is a water-soluble vitamin that helps the mother and baby to absorb iron and build a healthy immune system. It also helps the body to build tissue and hold cells together.

Pregnant women should consume at least 80-85 milligrams of Vitamin C per day. Nursing mothers should not consume any less than 120 milligrams of Vitamin C per day.

Vitamin C is an antioxidant that can be found in citrus fruits, raspberries, bell peppers, green beans, strawberries, papaya, potatoes, broccoli and tomatoes. It is also available in many cough drops and other supplements.

CALCIUM

Vitamin D is essential for building a baby's bones and may also promote optimal functioning of the baby's brain and heart.

Calcium is present in dairy products, such as milk, cheese, yoghurt and ice cream. It is also found in fortified juices and cereals. Vegetables like spinach, broccoli, okra, sweet potatoes, lentils and tofu contain calcium. Chinese cabbage, kale and broccoli are also good sources of this mineral. Calcium supplements are also widely available.To maintain healthy bones, pregnant women should consume at least 1200 milligrams of calcium a day and nursing mothers 1000 milligrams per day.

Calcium absorption is aided by Vitamin D, allowing both the mother and her child to develop healthy bones.

For optimal health during pregnancy and lactation, women should consume at least 2000 International Units (IU) of Vitamin D per day.

Babies require more Vitamin D than adults, and your doctor may recommend a vitamin supplement. Baby formula is also fortified with Vitamin D

Vitamin D deficiencies are usually corrected by taking supplements, but the vitamin can also be found in some foods such as milk, fortified cereals, eggs and fatty fish like salmon, catfish and mackerel. Vitamin D is also found in sunshine, so women and children found to have a mild Vitamin D deficiency may be told to spend more time in the sun.

VITAMIN D

Vitamin D improves the body's ability to absorb calcium, which leads to strong bones in both mother and child.

Pregnant or breastfeeding women should consume at least 2,000 IU of Vitamin D daily.

Although adults also need Vitamin D, babies require more of it. A doctor may recommend a supplement for an infant if her mother's milk does not provide enough nutrients she needs to grow.

Vitamin D is found in a few foods and must be supplemented through diet. Milk, cereal and eggs are among the best sources of fortified vitamin D; fatty fish like salmon, catfish and mackerel can also provide some dietary intake of this nutrient but may vary in content depending on location. People with low levels of Vitamin D in their blood may be advised to spend more time outside for sun exposure.

VITAMIN D

Vitamin E helps the baby's body to form and use its muscles and red blood cells.

Pregnant women should get at least 20 milligrams of Vitamin E daily, but no more than 540 milligrams.

Vitamin E is found in vegetable oil, wheat germ, nuts, spinach, and fortified cereals. It can also be taken in pill form.

It's better to get your Vitamin E from foods, like nuts, that are naturally high in nutrient than by taking synthetic supplements.

FOLIC ACID

Vitamin D improves the body's ability to absorb calcium, which leads to strong bones in both mother and child.

During pregnancy, folic acid is one of the most important vitamins. It plays an essential role in DNA replication, cell growth and tissue formation—all crucial for developing a healthy baby.

Folic acid deficiency during pregnancy can lead to birth defects such as spina bifida, anencephaly and encephalocele (an abnormal opening in the skull that allows brain tissue to protrude).

These conditions occur during the first trimester before most women know they're pregnant.

To ensure healthy fetal development, women should get enough folic acid before they conceive.

The recommended daily intake of folic acid for pregnant women is 0.6 to 0.8 mg per day.

Vitamin D improves the body's ability to absorb calcium, which leads to strong bones in both mother and child.

Folic acid is found in oranges, orange juice, strawberries and many other fruits and vegetables. It's also available as a supplement or added to some breakfast cereals.

IRON

This vitamin is essential for cell development, blood formation and placenta creation.

Pregnant women should have at least 27 mg of iron per day.

Iron is found in red meats, poultry, legumes (beans and lentils), vegetables, whole grains and fortified cereals.

NIACIN

It is known as Vitamin B3 and helps the mother's digestive system to function optimally, giving the baby energy for development.

For pregnant women, an intake of at least 18 mg of Niacin a day is recommended.

Niacin is found in many foods high in protein, such as eggs, meats and fish; it's also in whole grains, bread products and fortified cereals.

PROTEIN

Protein is the building block of all cells in the body. During pregnancy, when both Mom and baby are growing at a rapid pace, protein is especially important as it helps support cell growth.

Because of the extra demands, pregnancy and lactation place on a woman's body, pregnant and nursing women should consume at least 70 grams (about 25 more than the average nonpregnant/nonlactating woman needs) each day.

Protein can be found naturally in beans, poultry, red meats (beef), fish, shellfish and eggs. Milk products such as cheese or yoghurt also contain protein.

RIBOFLAVIN

Vitamin B2 is also known as riboflavin. It gives the body energy and helps develop a baby's bones, muscles and nervous system.

Riboflavin is important in the growth and development of fetuses, nursing babies, and infants.

Riboflavin is present in many foods, including whole grains, dairy products and meat.

THIAMIN

Thiamin, a form of Vitamin B1, helps the body develop important organs and central nervous system functions in babies.

Pregnant women, nursing mothers, and people with diabetes should take at least 1.4 mg of Thiamin daily.

Thiamin can be found in a variety of foods, including whole grain products, pigs' bodies (pork), fortified cereals made from wheat or rice and eggs.

ZINC

Zinc is vital to your fetus's growth because it aids in cell division, the primary process by which tiny tissues and organs grow. It also helps Mom and baby produce insulin as well as other enzymes.

Pregnant women should consume at least 11-12 mg of zinc daily.

Zinc can be found in red meats, poultry beans and nuts. It is also present in dairy products, fortified cereals and supplements for children who receive little or no animal protein during childhood.

NUTRITION AND EXERCISE ARE IMPORTANT DURING PREGNANCY

FITNESS AND NUTRITION DURING AND AFTER PREGNANCY

This chapter will explain the nutrition and exercise requirements for each trimester.

Now that you know what foods are best for pregnant women and how to stay active, everything should fall into place.

In this chapter, you will learn how to put into practice what you have learned about nutrition and eating well. You will also find detailed instructions for doing the exercises presented earlier in the book.

NUTRITION & EXERCISE DURING THE FIRST TRIMESTER

During your first trimester, you do not have to significantly increase the number of calories you eat. However, it is important that you get all the right vitamins and minerals, especially folic acid.

It is normal for pregnant women to gain weight during their first trimester. You should not try to diet; just enjoy the process of becoming a mother-to-be!

EXERCISE

The amount of exercise you can do during your first trimester will be determined by how strong and energetic you were before getting pregnant.

The mistaken belief that pregnant women should avoid exercise is unfounded. Indeed, pregnancy does not give you an excuse to become a couch potato, but it also doesn't mean you shouldn't be active during your term.

It is easier to stay healthy while pregnant if you are active; however, don't overdo it.

Do not engage in high-intensity workouts such as HIIT or Crossfit during your first trimester.

The best form of exercise is walking for a half hour every day. This can do wonders, both physically and emotionally. Have your partner join you so that exercising becomes something enjoyable instead of an obligation or chore.

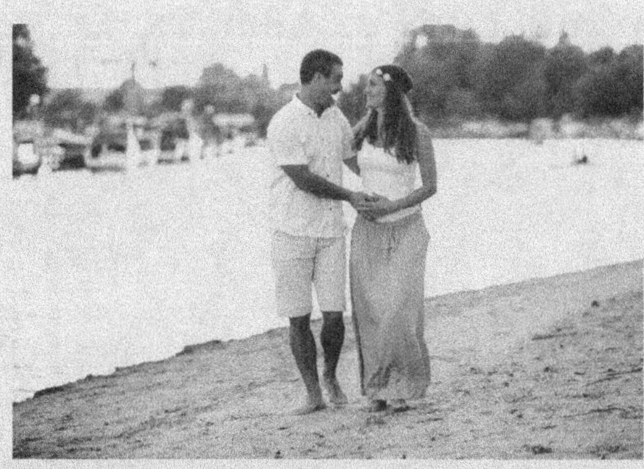

If you are accustomed to being physically active, you might find yourself in withdrawal if your workouts stop during pregnancy.

You may still participate in low-impact cardio workouts, such as riding a stationary bike.

Swimming is one of the best forms of exercise, because it is low impact and very effective.

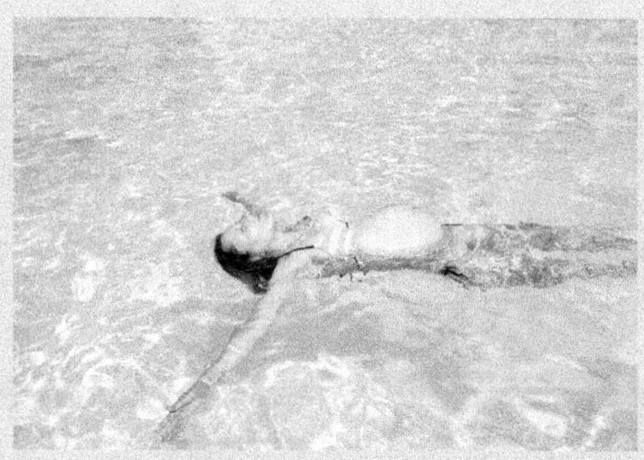

Exercises that cause your heart rate to increase rapidly should be avoided.

Do not exhaust yourself during your workout. Excessive breathlessness makes it difficult to maintain a consistent rhythm of movement.

Your goal with exercise is to enjoy the sensation of your blood pumping and to raise your heart rate. Don't push yourself too hard or you might get hurt—or discouraged!

A GUIDE TO HEALTHY EATING AND EXERCISE DURING YOUR SECOND TRIMESTER

NUTRITION

The food choices you make during each of the three trimesters will be the same. The only difference is that your calorie intake may vary from one to another.

You should add 300 calories to your daily diet during your second and third trimesters.

Your intake of calories should increase to compensate for the increasing rate of your baby's growth. If you were consuming 1800 calories pre-pregnancy, you should now be eating around 2100 a day.

If you consumed 1400 calories, then your body would burn 700 and store the rest as fat—a ratio of 2:1.

If you are eating more calories than your body burns, then of course you will gain weight.

It's fine for you to gain weight during pregnancy; don't worry about it.

It is normal to gain some weight during pregnancy. Eat the right foods and eat more so that there are enough calories and nutrients for your baby as well as for you.

EXERCISE

Unlike in the first trimester, most women experience fewer symptoms and feel more energetic during this stage of pregnancy.

A woman's energy level tends to rise during her second trimester.

That means you can enjoy more physical activity than previously possible. Of course, it is important not to strain yourself too much with high-impact exercises; however, when strength training, your muscles are used in various settings for maximal benefit.

The exercises that tone your back muscles, neck muscles and legs will be essential to maintaining good posture throughout pregnancy. Pregnancy strains all of these areas; many women notice aches in their backs or necks as they grow larger with a child.

The following exercises are some of the best moves to strengthen your body during pregnancy. If you do not know how to perform them, simply Google or YouTube the exercise and watch a video showing you how it's done.

- Squats

- Step ups

- Lunges

- Modified side planks

- Bird dog

- Bicep/triceps curls

- Straight Leg calf stretch

- Hip flexor stretch

You may continue with your walking or stationary bike workouts, though you will not be able to do any more than usual.

The way your body responds to exercise will vary from person to person.

Many women can continue exercising during pregnancy, especially if their doctor gives them the go-ahead.

Is this a good idea? That depends on you. Only you can know your own capabilities and limitations.

Physical contact, especially during competitive sports, can lead to the spread of infections and other diseases.

The best person to speak with about exercise is your doctor. He/she will be able give you advice on what types of exercises are most appropriate for your situation.

If you're healthy and have been active before pregnancy, chances are good that your routine won't need to change when you become pregnant.

You don't have to exercise just because you're now eating more calories than in the first trimester and might otherwise gain weight.

Mistreating a pregnant woman can affect her and the child she is carrying.

Enjoy your pregnancy. You will have the happy glow of a pregnant woman, and there is no need to worry about looking like a swimsuit model anyway!

NUTRITION AND EXERCISE DURING THE THIRD TRIMESTER

NUTRITION

It is important to have regular checkups with your doctor so that he/she can monitor your progress.

How many calories you need during the third trimester depends on how you feel. Your doctor will advise you if your diet needs adjusting. Just follow their recommendations by eating what they tell you to eat, and avoiding the things that they say not to.

EXERCISE

Your baby bump should show now, although it may make some exercise movements difficult. You can still walk or use a stationary bike.

The goal is simply to be active. Don't focus on your heart rate or sweating—it doesn't matter how hard you work. Just get up and move!

You can continue to perform the same strength-training exercises mentioned during your second trimester.

Alternatively, you may want to take a few classes in prenatal yoga. These classes focus on stretching and help relieve back pain, leg cramps and headaches many women experience during pregnancy.

During the last trimester, every movement might seem like an effort. If you feel that way during a prenatal exercise class, it's okay to take a break.

Being happy can help you, and your baby develop a strong bond.

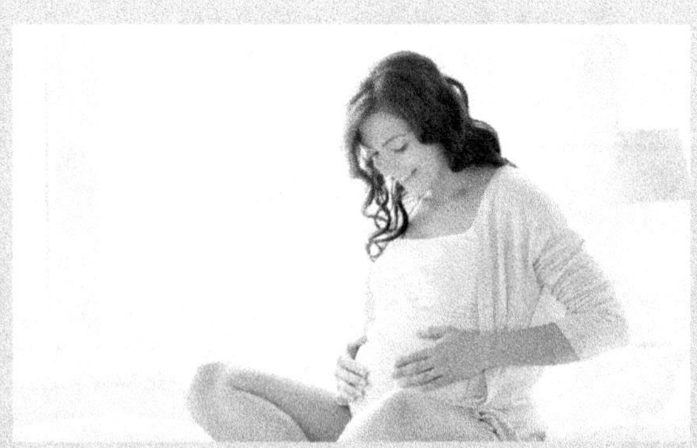

Meditating and relaxing to clear your mind and reduce stress is also a good idea. Research has shown that meditation boosts creativity, improves focus, increases endurance, makes your immune system stronger— and by extension, gets rid of colds faster!

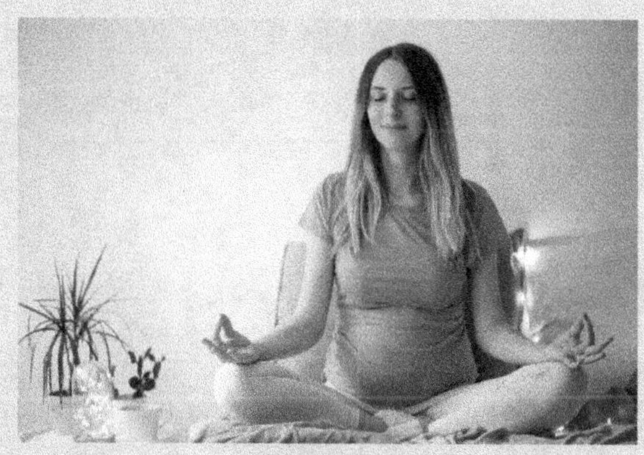

CHAPTER 6

YOU'VE FINALLY GOT YOUR BABY; WHAT COMES NEXT?

This is the part where you cuddle your baby and make cooing noises. It's also the part where, because you are recovering from childbirth, all of your partner's duties around the house for a short time fall onto his shoulders: like making sure we have enough diapers in stock (we don't), preparing meals he'll eat to be nice but never thinks about what I might want (breakfast after midnight?) , helping kids with their homework when they ask so that they can get it done without him having to hover over them or lose interest before finishing them or just not doing anything at all!

After childbirth, you may slowly reduce your calorie consumption. Continue to eat healthy and balanced meals so that your body can recover properly.

Breastfeeding your child will be one of the best things about pregnancy. But if you have any questions or concerns, feel free to discuss them with a physician.

There are a few important guidelines to keep in mind if you plan on breastfeeding your baby.

- It will hurt at first.
- Olive oil can be used to moisturize your nipples.
- Wear comfortable bras.
- Keep hydrated by drinking plenty of water.
- Eat well and get enough calories.

WHAT NEXT ?

Becoming a new mother is an ongoing process of learning. You can learn about this from books written for first-time mothers.

This book is concerned more with nutrition and fitness than weightlifting.

Let us now turn to how new mothers can regain their physical health.

You should wait two or three weeks after giving birth before beginning an exercise program.

You can now embark on a journey to achieve your dream body. To accomplish this, you must first get in shape.

You'll need to estimate how many calories your body burns each day to create the calorie deficit necessary for weight loss.

You should avoid cutting your calorie intake too low. This might make you feel like you're making progress, but it can slow down the rate at which your body burns fat.

After giving birth, you may feel ready to reclaim your old exercise habits. However, there are a few considerations that new moms should keep in mind.

It takes six weeks to three months for your body to return to its previous state after pregnancy.

That means that your workout should still be low-impact. Forget high-intensity interval training or sprinting: focus on low impact during workouts.

You will still lose weight at a steady rate, even if you weigh yourself daily. As long as your body is at a caloric deficit, losing fat and muscle mass cannot be stopped by weighing yourself every day.

If you walked for 30 minutes twice a day, your weight would decrease noticeably over time.

Want to challenge yourself? Walk up a steep hill. Want more of a challenge? Add ankle weights and walk uphill.

That's how you do it.

You can lose weight as long your diet is clean and healthy, you are at a caloric deficit each day.

For many women, losing weight is like trying to climb a mountain: it takes time and perseverance.

Do not give up on your weight loss goals just because you are having trouble losing weight. Time will pass whether or not you reach those goals.

If you do not make a conscious effort to improve, then in 8 months, you will remain where you are now.

Take a photo of yourself at the beginning, and then take one after six months or 1 year. You will see how much you have changed.

Most women can return to their pre-pregnancy body shape within six months if they work out, watch what they eat and do low-impact cardio daily.

If they can do it, so can you.

HOW TO MAXIMIZE YOUR FITNESS JOURNEY

FITNESS AND NUTRITION DURING AND AFTER PREGNANCY

After six months, talk to your doctor about increasing the intensity of your training program.

Once you get the go-ahead, take advantage of that opportunity.

Start training with weights and combine strength-building exercises with cardiovascular exercises.

Do short, intense cardio sessions instead of long ones. This will keep your body burning fat for hours after exercise.

In both cases, a caloric deficit and regular training are key.

To reach the highest levels of fitness is a matter of regularly performing demanding physical activities.

The more you train, the better your body will become. Three months of intense training is good. A year of it is great!

Mindset is also crucial.

A child's arrival is not a death sentence for your fitness.

In other words, nothing is stopping you from getting the body that you want. You are the only thing standing in your way.

Now you're a mother, and your child is watching what you do. Set a fitness goal for yourself!

Let your desire to achieve something become a goal in itself. Break the ultimate objective into measurable steps, and celebrate each as it is reached.

If you are patient and consistent, your dream body will be a reality before you know it.

People tend to take digs at others to make themselves feel better. It helps them overlook their own failings by making someone else appear imperfect.

You will also know that real success takes effort, discipline and determination —and isn't that the kind of person you want your child to be?

Of course, you do. They will learn more by watching what you do rather than listening to what you say, so be an example for the children—they'll one day look back and be proud of their mother.

Feeling fat is temporary, but being a mom and feeling proud of yourself will last a lifetime.